AN INTRODUCTION TO YOGA

Essential Yoga Poses That Will Help You to Achieve Inner Peace and Happiness

By ERIK FISHNER

Table of Contents

Introduction

The benefits of yoga are countless; much like the poses you can practice. I'm a novice yoga practitioner and believe in the advantages I've gained. I lost over one hundred pounds eating right and practicing yoga. It has allowed me to get healthy, feel better inside and have a more competitive edge than I ever thought possible. This book is intended for people that don't have a lot of time and want to get a maximum experience with minimal experience.

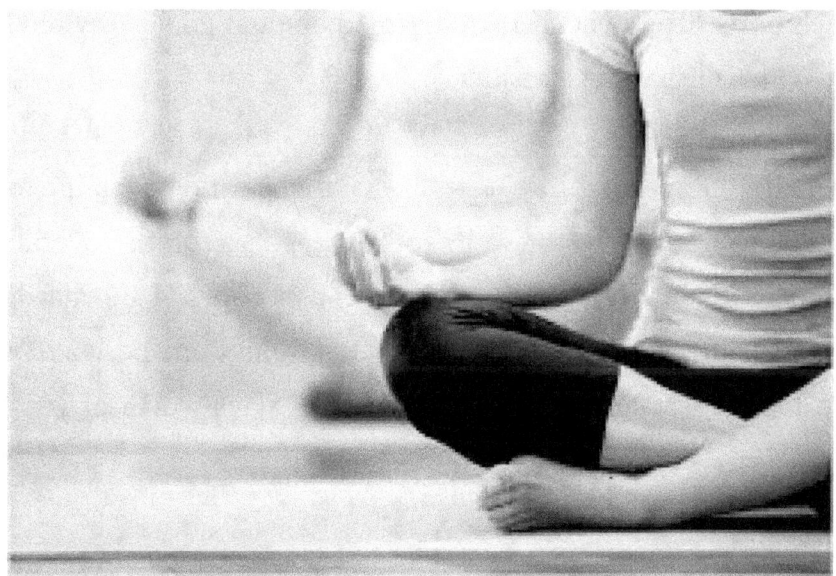

Instructions to the Reader:I lay no personal claim to these techniques or posing positions. The cumulated information and experience is something thatcan be researched either on the Internet or on your own. What I profess is how each of these poses benefitted me through the transition of being an overweight slug into a malleable man that isn't afraid to try something new if it will help me live a fulfilling and enriched life.

Always consult a physician before attempting any new exercises or lifestyle changes. Not everyone can do yoga and it will be a test of willpower, ligament stretching, and focused breathingthat will make the difference. Take your time, do as much or as little needed to achieve a personal goal every day. You will eventually see results.

It will not happen overnight. It takes patience and discipline to attain the desired results; either in the poses, or the overall practice. Listen to your body; don't push yourself too hard; especially in the beginning. Even if you attempt one pose a day that means you reached the goal of eight days worth of yoga poses.

Chapter 1: Looking Back and Gaining Wisdom

I was fat. I wasn't just fat, I was huge. There is something that happens internally when facing a weight issue. I knew that my blood pressure was increased. I understood that having high blood pressure leads to heart attack and strokes. I understood that having excess weight increased my chances of other medical problems. I knew all of that. I didn't need someone else reminding me that I was fat.

I knew I had distorted my self-image. Although I didn't own a mirror in the house that showed any part of my body below the shoulders; I took care when I looked in the bathroom mirror and made sure to not turn sideways. My clothing at home was loose fitting. I bought second-hand clothes that were XXL and sometimes XXXL. I thought it was okay to wear clothing with elastic waistbands around the house. However, I still had some sense of personal appearance when it came to leaving the house. I refused to wear running pants or sweatpants when I went shopping. My work appearance meant I had to wear a uniform.

I read somewhere that over 65% of obese people see themselves as overweight and not obese, and don't think they have a problem. I knew I had a problem. When I sat down and bent over to tie my shoes it was a struggle. I was winded during the simple procedure. My hands went numb every time I lay down to sleep. Sleeping was always a challenge. I had problems sleeping altogether. I figured it was stress from work. If I got more than four hours a night I thought that was enough. Then I would lay awake often until the alarm went off for work and I would get up. The bed groaned with relief every time. Since my sleep schedule was predictable, knowing I would get relatively 4 hours of sleep, I stayed up later. I watched television or read books until about one in the morning. The folly at that point meant since I was up later, I felt I needed to snack. Dinnertime was sometimes four to six hours earlier. I felt since I was awake anyway, why not have a snack?

I would eat potato or corn chips, cheese, and drink coffee until late in the night. I was under some impression that caffeine in coffee didn't affect me as it did others. I had the grand idea that I would drink coffee until 10 or eleven at night and when I was finally tired for bed around one or two in the morning, then any caffeine coursing through my body would either subside or urinated away before I lay down to sleep.

It wasn't just my sleeping patterns that were disrupted by poor diet, and terrible sleeping habits, my guts were suffering. I had severe Irritable Bowel Syndrome and constant burning in my chest from heartburn. Of course, eating chips or junk food in the middle of the night was affecting every other part of my body, not just my stomach. I was self-destructing and miserable. My attitude was bitter. I didn't know how poorly I treated other people around me. Something needed to happen.

I began feeling worse than normal. I felt IBS and heartburn were normal now. I never wore a coat when the weather got cold. I didn't feel cold like other people. I sweat most of the time inside and was moderately cool outside. Only under the most extreme cold did I feel a jacket was necessary. Even when I wore outwear, I didn't cover my head because it was the only way I could keep myself from sweating inside a coat. I never wore gloves. Since my hands were numb most of the time anyway, I didn't feel the chilly bite of winter weather in my fingertips.

With something else going on internally, I sought a medical opinion. I knew it was going to be expensive once I started going to see a doctor. I focused on the immediate changes in my health. I wasn't going to listen to someone tell me that I was overweight and I would feel better once I lost weight. I already knew that. I was always thinking of ways to lose weight. I thought starving myself throughout the day was the best course of action. Even to this day, after years of denying my body of food through the entire day, sometimes sixteen hours without food, my body is permanently scarred. When I found a doctor and began to visit her office, I was skeptical. I wanted to take some miracle prescription and that would quell the added misery; leaving me with my normal IBS and heartburn. Antacids and drinking generic bismuth sub-salicylate helped relieve enough of the symptoms so I could function through my business day. Once at home, if I spent a few hours sitting on the toilet, evacuating my fiery bowels, that was my business. By the time I finished in the bathroom most nights, I was unable to stand right away because I would lose all the feeling in my legs.

The doctor was versed in Homeopathy. Homeopathic cures have been in use alongside Western medicine for over three hundred years. A man named Samuel Hahnemann in 1796 decided to cure people with similar symptoms of existing diseases. What he learned was treating people with like symptoms. It's still considered a pseudoscience. Much like the manipulation of the human spine at the chiropractic clinic, real doctors, those employed at big hospitals and expensive private practices, feel Homeopathy has no place among the living. It's better living through the science of prescription medicine. Homeopathic medicine treated people psychological and not just the physical symptoms.

In a society that grew up watching pharmaceutical and medical commercials targeting people with severe to moderate hypochondria, any one of those commercials had, at least, three symptoms that I felt every day! Why not get on some prescribe medicine that aided my current painful symptoms?

I had no idea when I first went to this doctor's office that they specialized in Homeopathic procedures. She was recommended to me by a work colleague and I was lucky the doctor was still accepting new patients without referrals.

My first visit was routine, what I expected. Weight, blood pressure reading, and the doctor listening to me describe these new problems that were wreaking havoc with my insides. She was interested and patient and didn't suggest anything out of the ordinary. She didn't write me a prescription either. She suggested stop eating things with gluten. She said that would cure my newest ailments.

Two weeks later I returned to the doctor office for a follow-up and admitted her suggestion was valid. I had acquired a gluten allergy. I felt moderately better. I was almost back to my normal IBS and constant heartburn. I would have ceased going to her if I knew it was just that easy.
I learned from an anthropology class in college that since we were no longer hunters and gatherers, that we had access to

certain foods year around and not just when we seasonally collected them, that we were becoming dependent on certain foods that we once didn't eat. So grains and meats were no long separated by long winters and foraging summers. In the United States, we had constant access to anything we wanted to eat, anytime we want. The local grocery store has tons of food always available. There were fresh foods and foods so full of preservatives they had a half life and not just a shelf life. I learned quickly that locating foods free of gluten weren't only difficult it was also more expensive. It is a strange realization that comparing the ingredients in a candy bar and that of a cauliflower that a candy bar cost less than a head of cauliflower! Junk food taste better than cauliflower! Also, a head of cauliflower tastes better when it's smothered in some blue cheese. Unfortunately, most blue cheese dressing and vegetable dips had gluten.

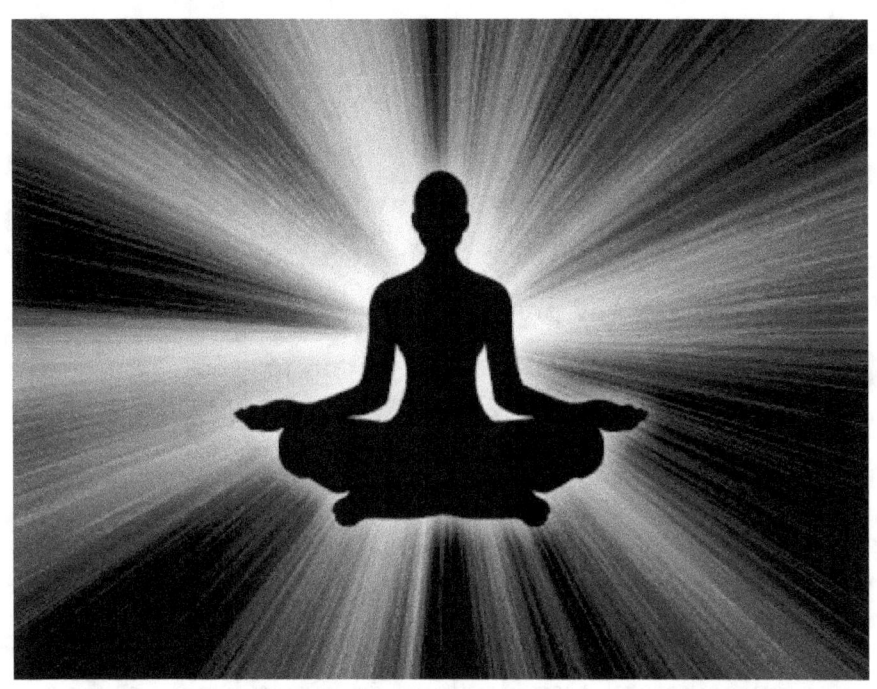

The doctor suggested that I should consider some exercise program. Since I knew it was coming, I felt I would rebuff her suggestion by pointing out that I already exercised all day, every day. I worked long hours and was on my feet all day; I walked several miles a day inside the business. Wasn't that exercising enough? I was on a fixed budget. A membership to the local gymnasium was out of the question. I couldn't afford that extra expense.

The doctor was experienced with resistance. She made a living in an industry that fed off the medically insured populous and ignored people without healthcare plans. She understood a fixed budget and worked her office patients on a sliding scale.

Sometimes she accepted people without healthcare and did everything in her power, often her back against the rest of the medical world, to help people less fortunate than an overweight, middle-class Caucasian male. I would say that she was passive aggressive, but she actively listened to my complaints about my problematic body, and would point out that my symptoms followed a certain pattern, much like smaller satellites circling larger universal bodies, my internal problems revolved around my obesity.

She asked me to think about it, to consider what I was willing to do to make myself feel better. She asked me to change one thing immediately: stop drinking so much coffee; especially after six at night.

What bought this distinct fact that I was obese directly in my face was when I got sized for a pair of slacks for work. When the seam split on one of my work slacks, I knew I had to buy another pair. I went to a local shop that sold specific clothing for my employment. I told the female attendant that I needed a size 40" waist pair of slacks.

She returned with the pants I thought I needed. She asked if I was going to try on the slacks before I left the store. I had never tried on a pair of pants at a store before. I never saw the reason in it. Every pair of slacks within a given waist size and length were identical. Why waste my time putting on clothes that I already knew would fit fine?

Since she seemed sincere I shrugged and went to the changing room. There was a full-length mirror inside the little closet that I attempted to ignore as much as I could. The slacks she tried to sell me were the wrong size. That is to say, they were labeled size 40" waist and the proper length, but I couldn't climb into them all the way. There was a considerable difference from the size 40" pants that I wore to the shop, and the pair of slacks I needed for work.

I explained there must have been a mistake with the manufacturer. She smiled at me in a way that wasn't condescending. She genuinely must have experienced that sort of reaction from potential customers all day at the retail outfit. She grabbed a tape measure and wrapped it around my waist, made a mental note, and disappeared into the backroom. The pair of slacks she brought back to me not only fit but unlike the pants I wore to the shop, I was not stuffed into and hanging over the belt buckle. I was immediately depressed and left the shop with a realization that I had been in denial for far too long. Defeated, I returned to the doctor's office with one agenda, I needed to make serious changes to not only my diet but every aspect of my life if I wanted to continue to live longer and healthier.

The doctor understood my plea. She was empathetic to my problems. I weighed close to three hundred pounds, and my health was failing. Since I was open to committing to a better lifestyle, she was ready to offer me a solution. "Have you ever considered yoga?"

Chapter 2: Chaos and Order

Making drastic changes in my life to make room for something else took a lot of effort. It wasn't just wrapping my head around yoga; I had to find time to commit to the practice of the art and meditation practices that made up the yoga. My day was already overloaded with work and resting. If I wasn't on my feet all day long at work, I rested my aching feet at home, sprawled on the couch. Since I had already committed to not drinking coffee after 6 pm, I found there were more hours in the night for sleep. Although the sleep opportunity was intermittent, still restless, there was more night leftover when I woke from dosing to gain a few more hours of the precious night before I started another long day.

I realized if I was going to include one more activity in my life I had to make room in my schedule, and my house for the proper embrace of the lifestyle changes. It began with reading about something that I knew absolutely nothing about.

Part 1: History

Considering that I would do something I knew nothing about isn't so challenging to me as it might be for others. I consider myself fortunate that I am willing to try something new; especially if it will benefit me in the end. I began reading on the Internet about the history of yoga and how it has evolved since it began.

The history is a little convoluted. Much like certain religious practices, there are differing opinions about the birth of yoga and where it originates. One thing came clear is how yoga was part of a meditation practice. It didn't matter to me where it started, which culture wanted to lay claim to its origin. It mattered to me how the practice of yoga was going to work for me.

The "spiritual discipline" of yoga is a human evolutionary experience that came from the ancient Middle Eastern study of mind and body. Hinduism, Buddhism, and Jainism all have roots that carry yoga practices. Each of the cultures proudly carries their heritage arts into the modern age from 1700 to 500 BCE. That is a considerably long time to practice something, hand it down from generation to generation, along with scriptures and practical experiences. One would think that the art of yoga would have finally been mastered by someone by now.

Part2: Then and Now and Doing

Having a basic idea of what I was getting myself into meant I was generalizing the practice. If I was going to start doing yoga I was going to do it right. I wasn't going to just practice it; I was going to master it! I was going to streamline the procedures and do what I needed to do in half the as everyone else doing yoga.

When I was growing up the clothing industry began making baggy clothing. Youth culture wanted to rebel against their strict parents and the clothing that they were forced to wear. New styles of clothing began to immerse the society in a nation of young people that not only didn't want to wear belts; they didn't want to wear clothes that fit them accordingly.

While I fought obesity and had to contend with pants that were always too tight because of an expanded waistline, the youth around me wore pants that were so large they had to carry them in fists to wear. What was the point of this? I guess in my aged eye, clothing should be worn without having to hold them up with your hands. Wear a belt; leave your hands free for something else.

Slowly the clothing industry has changed. Young people are wearing clothes that are fitting their thin hips and even tight enough to still wear without belts. Recently, lawmakers in Montana want to outlaw yoga pants. It was the same when young people wore overtly bagging pants; there were fuddy-duddy lawmakers that wanted to ban baggy pants as well. At least now young people can keep their pants around their waists. Unfortunately, at the risk of outlining any embarrassing bodily features, yoga pants were completely out of the question for my physic.

Consider what you want to achieve when you begin with yoga. One important part of practicing poses is to not just getting your body into a pretzel shape, you need to mentally practice yoga. That means to make sure when you are ready to begin, you do it without distraction.

If you have a demanding life that includes children, spouses, and pets, you will likely not have an open space to practice yoga. If the children don't interrupt you, the pets will likely want to know why you are suddenly on the floor with them; if not to play.

I know people that have such a busy life at home, the only quiet place they have is in the bathroom. Unless you have a bathroom large enough to practice yoga, at least, attempt to close yourself off from the immediate world so you can have a few minutes to focus on yourself.

I don't recommend practicing yoga in your car driving back and forth from work. However, you can practice breathing while you drive. I know sometimes to wind down at the end of the day, I will find myself breathing and counting, the same practice you will learn later in this book.

Breathing is very important in yoga. Even if you can't get a rhythm immediately that you can maintain, you will eventually reach a momentum in your breathing that will allow your body to expand and contract as needed with each position.

Part3: Procrastination the Patient Killer

Taking the time to get off the couch once I was home for work was the most difficult, and painful thing to overcome with the embrace of yoga. I had to teach myself daily that I needed to do something more than just kick off my work shoes and plan my expanding behind on the couch. I had to overcome the idea that I needed to rest. My body told me often that it was tired, that it was sore. I had to convince my aching limbs, back, and feet, that if I took a little more time in my day before I sat down on the couch to rest my weary bones, it would actually be a good thing.

This is easier to mentally say than do. I suspect people making lifestyle changes all go through this procrastination period. I didn't just change overnight. The act of performing yoga for the benefit of my body and soul took weeks to actually happen.

17

I would lie on the couch after work, or wake up in the middle of the night, and think that I had to do something to stop feeling so bad. If I was going to master this yoga thing it, I had to actually start doing yoga! I had to take steps to make things happen if I was going to lose weight, and have the energy to do yoga.

Making life changes is a sometimes painful. Having the energy to make those changes that will benefit your body, your soul, and those people in your paradigm is a journey unto itself. I took steps to make things happen and stopped procrastinating.

Chapter 3: 8 Basic Yoga Poses to Change Your Life

The first real step to yoga begins on the floor. It doesn't matter if you go to a specific location that offers yoga classes, or you are like me and just find a quiet, open area in your home that offers you a free space for the poses, you will start on the floor.

Protect your knees! I cannot stress this enough. In my line of work, I have to be up and down on my knees. When you're young, twenty-something, you don't consider the future health of your knees an important factor in your lifestyle. However, anyone that has a weight problem, or has trauma to the legs, will tell you the same thing: protect your knees.

The first pose in basic yoga is just to sit on the floor. It may sound strange, but if you can sit on the floor comfortably, and get up again, you have already achieved, possibly mastered the first pose in yoga.

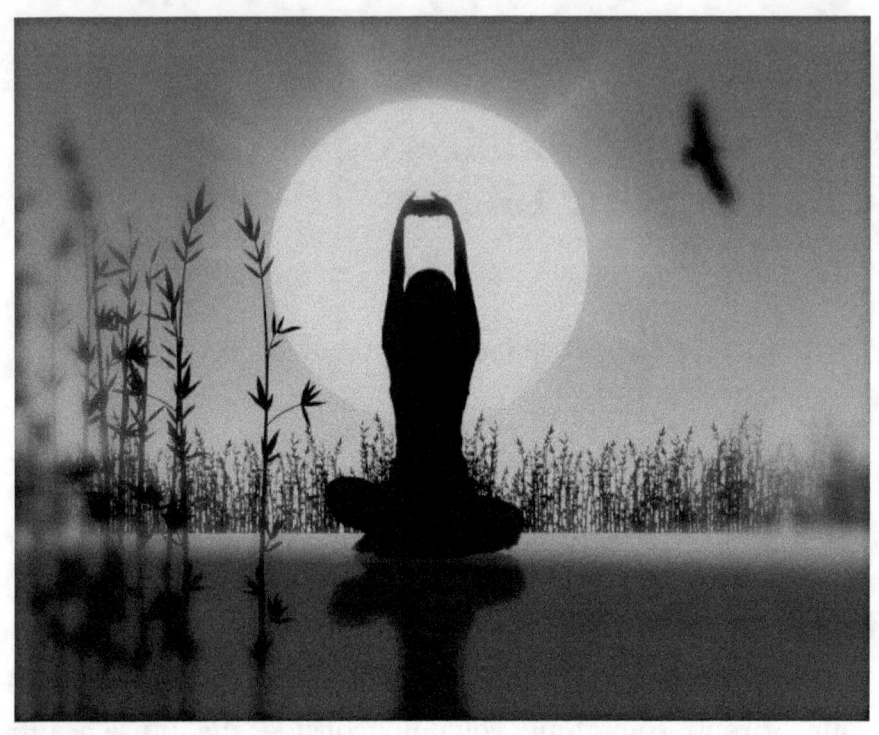

As a child, I spent hours lying or sitting on the floor. When you are practicing yoga it is important that you are not sitting on a hard surface. Spend a little money and buy a yoga mat. Make sure when you are ready to sit down on that mat you are wearing comfortable clothes. If you are in the privacy of your own home, wear something that breathes and stretches. I suggest you don't go out and buy a new yoga wardrobe. It would benefit you to have a pair of sneakers that have a rubber sole and are laced tight. Make sure the sneakers you wear have arch support for your feet. Don't wear any footwear that doesn't feel natural.

If you decide to forgo the footwear, at least, make sure you don't wear socks that can slip on a smooth surface. Often I see people that are barefoot. I choose to wear a pair of sneakers that have a strong arch support and are laced tight. Much like your wardrobe, your shoes are your business.

The act of sitting on the floor (or on a yoga mat) will require some discipline. You need to consider actually getting to the floor in a manner that is comfortable. This needs to be repeated when you get up again. Consider practicing getting down on the floor and back up again as a basic step to mastering yoga. As children, we started out crawling on the floor. This act of yoga posing will make the rest easier to accomplish.

Once you are on the floor, either sit on your feet, knees together. Or sit cross-legged. I have some dexterity leftover from my childhood. Since I have joint mice or loose fragments that float within the synovial space between my skin and patella, I choose to sit cross-legged. If I can keep away from direct contact with the floor and my kneecaps, I will have a better day.

The act of sitting comfortably on the floor comes not only in sitting there. It is an important process that will help you evolve spiritually and physically. It may sound strange, but eventually, you will look forward to a place of solace (other than sleep) that you can have a few minutes to breathe, and unwinding accordingly.

When you found your perfect beginning position, either sitting on your feet or cross-legged, you can begin practicing breathing. It is important to remember to take a position that is both comfortable and symmetrical. Humans are designed in a way that allows you a balanced body. Of course, not everyone is perfect. I know when I started, sitting cross-legged on the floor, I could feel my big Buddha belly touching my thighs. Let me tell you, that was discouraging. When you know you have that much surplus on your body that you can feel it hanging heavily on your thighs, it was further motivation to get rid of the weight.

Once you achieve that comfortable symmetrical pose, you must breathe accordingly. When you read about yoga you will see some authors devote chapters to just breathing! Learning how to breathe shouldn't be that difficult. After all, you've been doing it since birth! How difficult is it to just breathe?

Much like the benefit of breathing out or expelling air when you work with free weights, pressing a heavy weight away from your body, the act of breathing out properly during yoga will allow your lungs to strengthen while you work on the poses.

Breathing is vital to your body and especially your brain. Controlling your breathing to help you focus on yoga poses will be easier as you practice. Acquiring the right breathing technique will allow your body to increase blood flow and allow the posing in yoga to exercise all of your body. That intake of air is as important as letting out that air. Each breath we exhale has toxins that your body is always trying to get rid of.

You are seated comfortably on the floor (yoga mat or rug) and you are now focusing on breathing properly. Hopefully, there are no distractions. You can focus on breathing properly. From this point forward when you are breathing during the eight yoga poses, you will subconsciously know how to breathe properly. Breathing properly during yoga allows you the full benefit of each pose.

Although there are several techniques to breathing, much like yoga poses. It is important for a beginner to just focus on what is right for you. Consider that breathing and sitting are synonymous with each other. The moment you consciously think about doing yoga, you should subconsciously be practicing breathing. This premeditated understanding of breathing will come as easily as, well, *breathing*.

We breathe in a manner that is subconscious. We just do it. We don't have to think about breathing, it is part of our genetic makeup. Without breathing, well I don't have to tell you what happens next. What you need to think about when you're breathing is how your body wants to do it.

When you are focusing on your breathing something wonderful happens. You begin to consider how your body is working. Here you are sitting on the floor in a very relaxed manner, and now you are considering how your body is taking in and getting rid of air.

Our lungs are dependent on the diaphragm. The diaphragm forces the lungs to expand and contract. Your lungs are just empty sacs that would just remain immobile without the diaphragm moving them. When you breathe with yoga, at least as a beginner, you are taking steps to focus on how your diaphragm works.

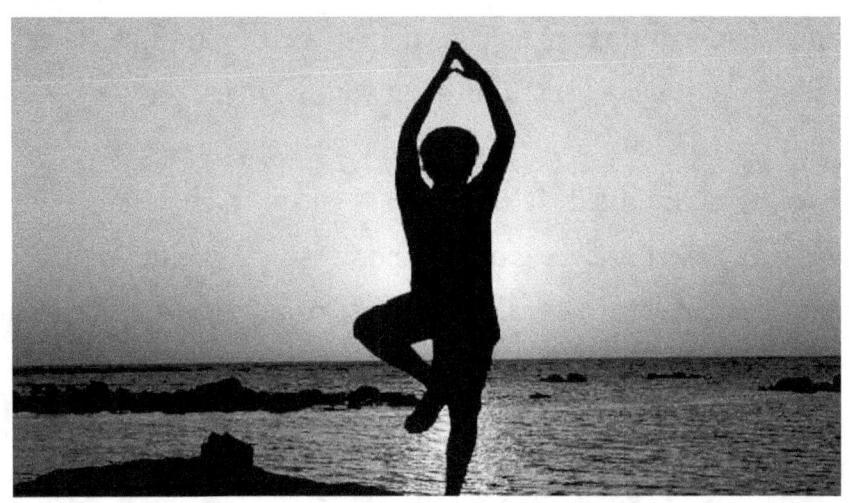

If you have been doing this since you sat on the floor, you are already well on your way to mastering yoga. The breathing is a big part of meditation, exercise, and concentration. There are plethoras of breathing techniques that will allow you to achieve some remarkable things. However, for the beginner yoga practitioner, a 3-part breathing practice will suffice.

Practice breathing in the upper chest. Often you will feel your belly doing all the work that your lungs should be doing. When you breathe using your belly, you miss out on the benefit of a large lungful of air. Having that extra bit of air that you have been missing out will begin working immediately.

Taking a deep breath, focusing on upper chest breathing will about your lungs full expansion, and immediately your body will thank you for a deep breath of clean air. What's interesting is how you can further help your body getting that clear air is taking in that deep breath through your nostrils.

Your nose is filled with filters. Those pesky hairs that eventually start crawling out of the nostrils of aging men, and some women, are natural filters that trap particles in the air before they can get to your lungs and contaminate your body.

Take a deep, closed mouth breath, using the upper chest. And hold it for a moment. When you release that lungful of air, expel it through your open mouth. It is important to consider your state of being at this point. Many people will feel lightheaded when you begin breathing in yoga. That is your body's way to tell you to relax and consider what you are doing. It does not benefit you if you are trying too hard, too fast. Take your time and breathe in a manner that allows you the full benefit of the breathing technique without overwhelming yourself, getting lightheaded, and possibly passing out. At least, if you are starting out seated on the floor, you won't fall far if you happen to pass out.

The object of the breathing is to allow your body to experience something new. Ease into it and take your time. If you experience any tension or lightheadedness, consider how you are breathing and make modifications that allow you to receive the full experience without discomfort. When I started out I got dizzy a lot. I learned quickly that proper breathing allowed me to feel better, I felt my body begin to relax, and I found that the beginning of my yoga practice was about fifteen minutes of just learning how to sit still on the floor and breathe in a manner that didn't make me want to pass out.

You can get lists of how many breaths to take, and how long each of these poses should take you. However, what I learned in practicing yoga, much like time, it is relative to the observer.

Chapter 4: Cat-Cow (Silly Little Things)

This part of the yoga poses requires some fortitude and faith. If you're like me and have some complications with your knees, it may not work for you. There are other alternatives that can be used as a substitute. However, what I've learned is how the body will adapt to certain parameters and if you take some care and precautions when you begin this part of your yoga poses, you will eventually feel that it isn't as impossible as you first suspected.

Considering that you are already on the floor, or yoga mat, getting into this position should be relatively easy. Just remember that you are getting into bodily positions that for most of us haven't tried since before we could walk upright.

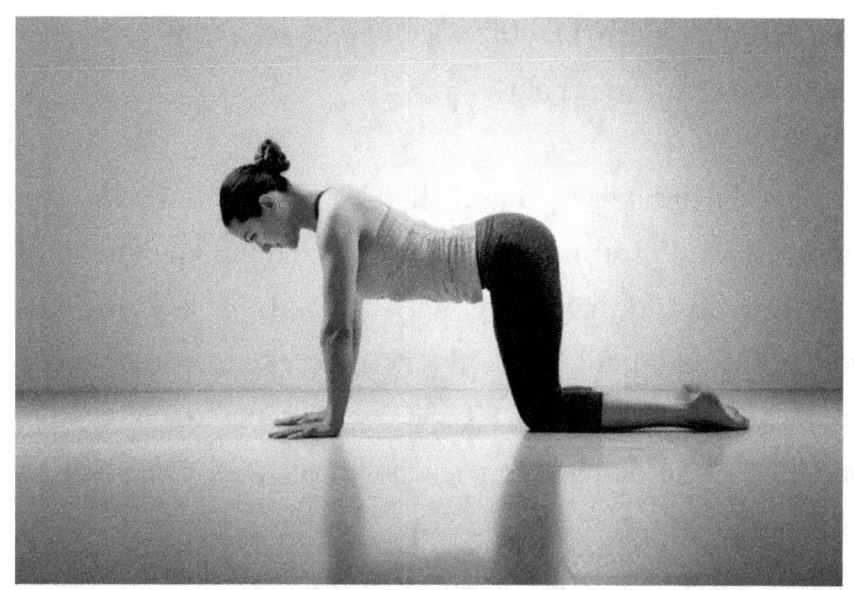

This is relatively easy if you have the ability to get on your hands and knees. You can rest as much as needed to achieve this part of the exercise. Just take your time and relax. Most exercise routines are 20-minutes in length, from beginning to end.

However, you will find that yoga is not exactly a timed routine. You can take as long or as short amount of time for each of the following poses.

For Cat-Cow posing, just remember to protect those knees. Once you are on all fours breathe as you've already practiced. Take air in through your nose and exhale slowly through your mouth. With each breath, you should focus on using your chest instead of your belly.

In the beginning, I found that my belly muscles were nonexistent. I'm sure there were some abdominal muscles but they were lost to time and gravity. I found that as I was on all fours, my belly hung to the floor. Hopefully, not touching the floor as you practice the Cat-Cow. Bracing the abdominal muscles while doing this yoga pose will take discipline and concentration. It will have a significant effect on the abdominals as you practice the Cat-Cow.

Stretch your spine slowly, and turn your head to face the ceiling. As you do this you will find that your body naturally arches the spine. You achieve a U-shape while facing the ceiling. Maintain this posture for approximately 30-seconds.

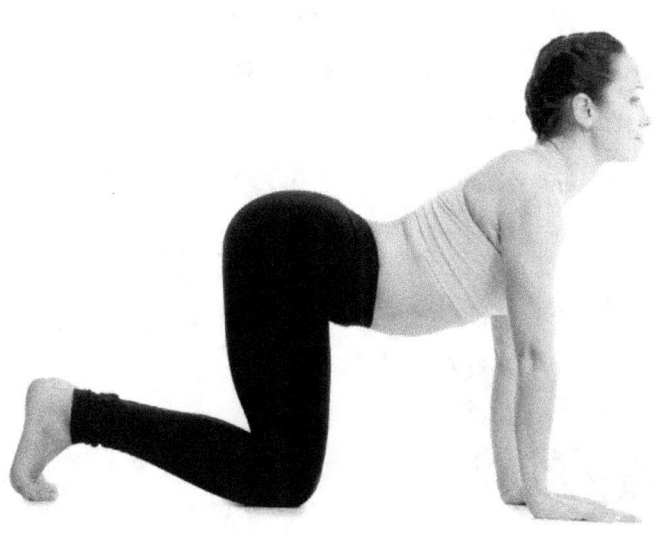

When you are ready, exhale and lower your head down. Continue to lower your head so your chin touches your chest. Simultaneously arch your back like a "cat" and hold that position for approximately 30-seconds.

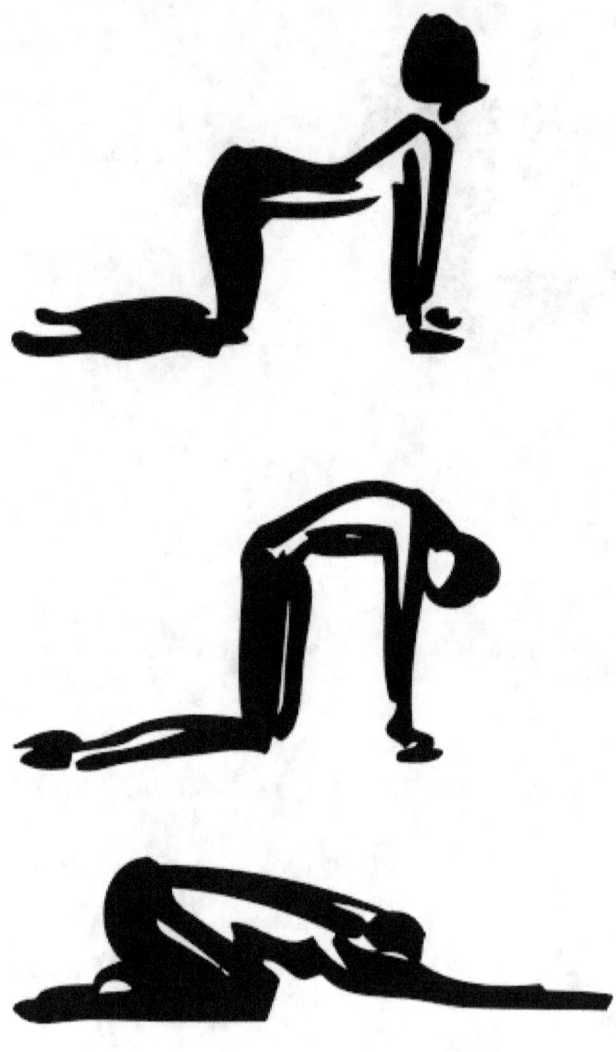

Continue to alternate this position from raised head, back U-shaped, to lowered head, back arched. Each time you do these continue to breathe and feel the full extending of your spine. I found when I started to do this my back groaned some. I felt some tension in my lower back. Before I began doing these yoga poses I learned it was best to stretch every available muscle. Much like going to the gymnasium, you will need to limber up before beginning yoga.

Take as long as you need for the Cat-Cow. However, I recommend that you give it a chance to work your spine, from head to tail. It will take some time before your body warms up to this. You will find that as you work your muscles, you will be able to hold these poses longer.

Chapter 5: Downward Dog (Animal Matters)

Anyone with house pets, cats, and dogs, know they spend a considerable amount of time sleeping. After hours of lying lazily around the house waiting patiently for you to come home, they will get up and stretch before they really start galloping around.

The common dog has a certain stretching technique that benefits the entire torso and limbs. This pose will take a little longer to learn and master than the Cat-Cow, but the Downward Dog has a lot of benefit for your entire wellbeing.

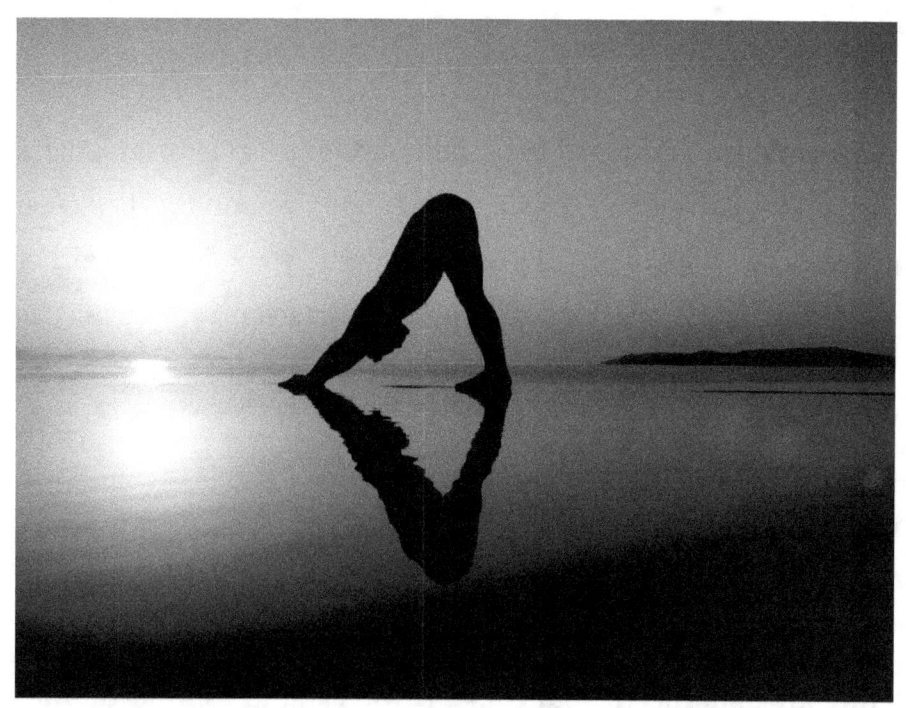

Since you are in the Cat-Cow pose, and likely a little out of breath, take your time and maintain contact with the mat. Hands flat against the floor, raise your knees off the mat. You will need to lift your buttock up, as you do this pose you will find a point where you are comfortable.

What you are going to eventually achieve is to have your derrière higher than your head. You want to have your feet flat on the floor. This will not be easy. If you are unable to get your feet flat on the floor, you can attempt to stretch while on the balls of your feet. However, it is important that you are in a position that will not cause you to slip.

Yoga mats are designed to be skid resistant. Nonetheless, there is potential for slippage. Make sure when you do this pose you are secure with your surroundings and your feet are either barefoot or you are wearing proper slip-resistant sneakers. The Downward Dog will take your breath away. Just remember to breathe and take your time.

As you exhale and raise your buttock to the ceiling, your hands should be on the mat, feet on the floor and your hips are in line with your shoulders. Keep your head down, face the floor directly underneath your torso. If you can dip your head lower and look at your stomach you are going to benefit even more from this pose.

The goal of this exercise is to create a straight line with your spine; position that allows your body to maintain an upside down V-shape. It will help your stretch if you remember to breathe deep, upper chest breathing. And attempt to deepen the postural with each exhale. If you can hold this position, breathing accordingly for at least one minute, you will find it will invigorate you and really help stretch those back muscles.

What's interesting about the Downward Dog is how your body already wants to tighten the abdominals. Your stomach will likely be sore for a short time after this because if you are like me, you haven't used your stomach muscles like this for a very long time.

Chapter 6: The Warrior Pose (Kung-Fu You)

I love old Chinese kung fu movies. What I noticed about this next pose was how many of the action film stars would position themselves in the Warrior's Pose either at the beginning of their battle or at the end for dramatic effect.

This pose begins with standing. If you are doing these in the order they appear in this book you are likely ready to stand up again. Remember: protect those knees. I learned that after I lost a lot of weight I still had problems with my knees. Substantial weight loss caused a lot of joint pain, especially in my knees. People that go to the gym and do high-impact exercising can cause considerable harm to their joints if they are heavy when they start out. Yoga is a low impact exercise and not as stressful on the joints.

I learned that as I lost a lot of weight, my knees hurt worse than they did when I was heavy. Apparently that added cushion in the knees helped naturally absorb the shock of just walking around. When the weight dropped off, the padding at the knees went with it.

There are a few variations of this particular pose. The first phase, the easiest phase, I will call simply the Warrior. The other variations of this yoga pose can be found across the Internet if you want to challenge yourself. For the benefit of maintaining introductory ideals, this will allow your body to understand what you want to obtain, and possibly grow with as you continue to use yoga for inner peace and stress management.

Start by spreading your feet out. Attempt to get a full opening with your legs without losing your balance. You will need to remember that you will be turning once your feet are spread apart, so maintain a posture that will keep you balanced. Once you do this pose a few times you will get an extended depth with your legs apart.

Start with your right side. Turn your right foot so it is line with your right shoulder, your arms stretched parallel with the floor. Your left foot will naturally fall into a place that allows you to keep your upright balance. Keeping your shoulders relaxed and your arms outstretched with your palms facing down, you have the beginning of the pose.

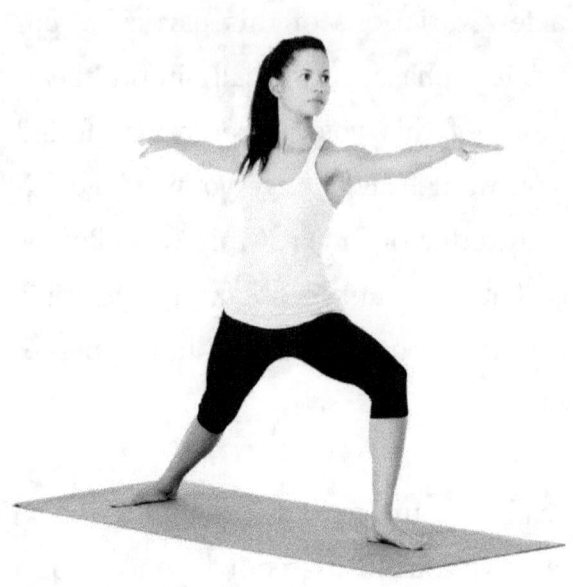

Now slowly bend your right knee. You want to have your knee straight over the toes of the right foot. If you try to push your knee further than your toes, you can hyperextend and create some problems in your thighs and back.

Stretch and hold for as long as you can and breathe with your upper chest. Once you feel you have this pose, then turn and do the same with your left side. Remember to walk or slide into it. If you try to just turn left, you will lose your balance. One thing about yoga that I learned as I do these poses is how your mind gets focused on the routine. Time just slips by and by the end I feel refreshed and focused.

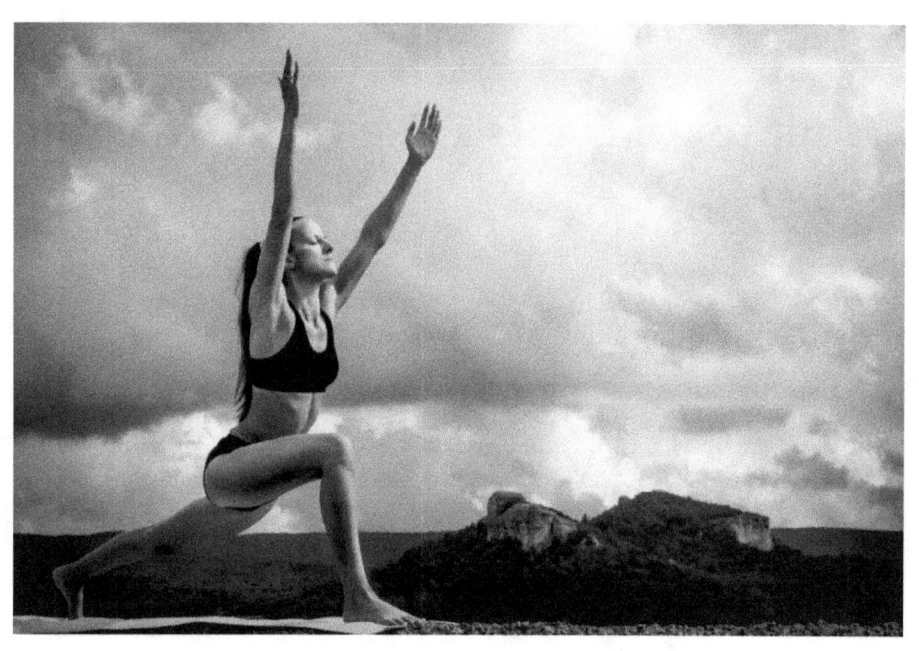

Chapter 7: Chair Pose (The Invisible Seat)

The Chair Pose is much like it sounds, just without the chair. It is a simple idea and will really have an impact on your thighs. This yoga pose helps me with balance and stability while increasing the strength in my legs. Although I am on my feet for sometimes fourteen hours in a day, my legs are used to moving a certain way. I can walk ten miles in one day, but it is a natural repetitious movement that your legs are very accustomed to doing in life. When you ask your body to change up its routine, you will find there are parts of your calf and thigh muscles that will fight against the change.

When you attain this pose correctly you will feel the isometric design within the human body that allows a natural curvature of the spine to maintain while the muscles that run along the spine, the erector muscles, to strengthen and will develop over time as you continue to do these exercises.

I found that as I did this exercise I felt some tension in my back muscles. I wanted to stop, but I felt that I needed to just figure out what my particular natural pose was when I sat in the invisible chair. Eventually, I learned that the natural curvature of my spine allowed me more arch in my back. Where the other exercises want you to stretch your back straight, this yoga pose wants you to achieve a balance within your posture that allows you to hover over the floor. Think of the pose you obtain when you are about to sit in a chair, and freeze.

Getting started is as natural as standing erect. Your feet should be shoulder width apart and straight ahead. So if you are standing natural, your feet are aligned with your hips. You lengthen your spine by raising your arms over your head. If you inhale as your do this, using the upper chest breathing you will feel your spine stretch.

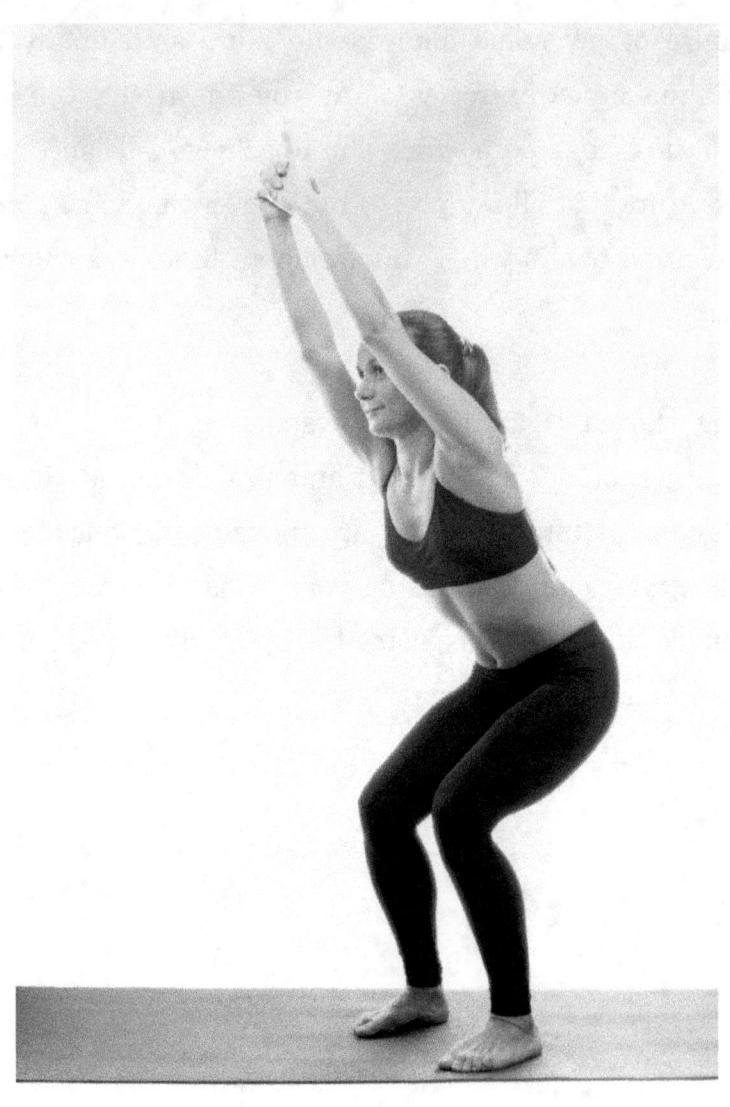

Normally when you bend over your spine curves and your body creates a hunch. When you do the Chair Pose correctly, your spine will be straight as you bend your hips forward. Keep your arms stretched out, palms down toward the floor and lean forward until you are at a 45-degree angle. Don't bother worrying too much if you get this pose or the angle correctly. If you do it and feel the impact, you will still get the benefit from the Chair Pose. Lower your upper body forward, maintaining that straightness in your spine until you reach (approximately) 45-degrees.

Now bend your knees as if you are ready to sit down on that invisible chair. The object is to keep the pose without losing your balance. If you feel you are concentrating too much on maintaining the angle, then you are losing the benefit of the Chair Pose because you cannot fully appreciate the yoga maneuver. Attempt to hold that pose, arms outstretched and breathing.

Pressing your bottom to the floor and slightly arching your back will allow you to come to a more natural pose and hold it. If you are breathing right, you will feel your abdominal muscles pulling as you achieve a pose that allows your tailbone to come to rest, hovering directly over your feet.

If you are comfortable doing this pose, you can deepen your seat, press your weight further to the floor. It becomes harder the deeper you stretch your thighs and bend your knees. If you come to a squatting position, you likely have gone too far into the Chair Pose. The idea is to sit in the air. However, I am not one to judge, if it feels good to make your thighs and knees work, then do it. There is no right way or wrong way to do a yoga pose unless you are performing something impossible on YouTube or have worked in acrobatics. If you are that limber and can bend without causing damage, tearing muscles, that is great!

Chapter 8: Upward Facing Dog (Looking Up)

This yoga pose is one of the iconic poses you see on countless websites. It has a lot of benefit for your body, muscles and circulation. It feels great and really stretches your muscles.

Much like the title suggests, and reminiscent of the Downward Dog, your pets do this kind of thing every time they wake from a nap. However, it is important to know what feels right when you practice this pose. If you do something that doesn't work well with your body, align symmetrically, you will feel discomfort.

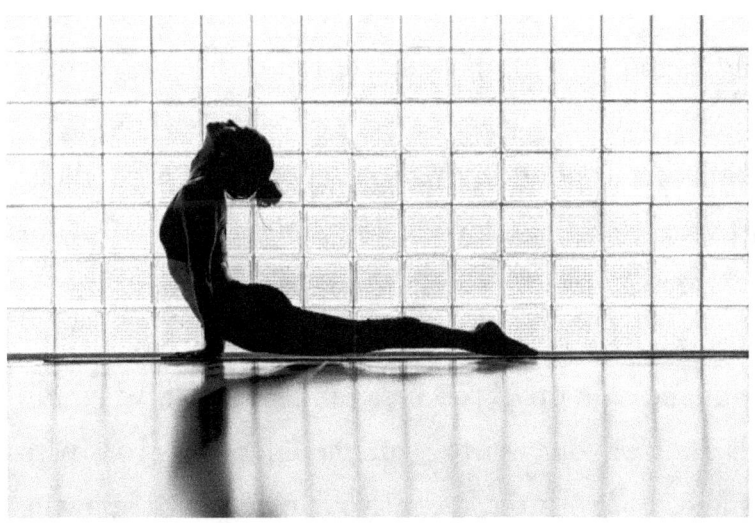

What's really important with this particular pose is how you distribute your weight across the floor mat. You want to make sure you don't put too much weight on your wrists, especially if you haven't done this pose before or may not be used to feeling how much you weigh through your hands.

Focus on what you are trying to do with this pose. The right alignment of your core will allow you to know immediately if you are performing this right or wrong. The real challenge with this pose is how you naturally want to allow your body weight to fall to the floor. The more of your body weight on the floor, the less you have to lift and hold. The proper posture of this pose forces you to consider what your shoulders are doing while you practice. You don't want to allow your shoulders to roll forward. That is a nature reaction to the tension you put on your body as you do this pose. When you put too much weight on your wrists, your body compensates by using your shoulders to help with the burden.

The other focus point in this pose is how you press the tops of your feet into the mat. If you allow your body to fall against the mat, you will feel the weight pressuring your lower spine because your pelvis will drop to the mat. Keep your head straight and chin up. If you press and hold your weight in your hands and not your wrists, your shoulders will work with your arms and, not with the rest of your core; fighting against the strength of your arms. You should feel your shoulder blades working on your back, and if they want to pop out, then you are misaligned.

Instead of allowing your thighs to rest on the mat after you have reached the position, you want to actively use the top of your feet to lift your knees off the mat. You will feel this pressure in your quadriceps. If you can maintain this pose you will feel the pressure in your thighs and calf muscles. You are distributing your weight across the plane of your body just above the floor. The back will arch in a manner that you allow by maintaining your shoulders, keeping them from rounding forward and the weight of your body in the palm of your hands and not in the wrists.

When you reach this pose, you will see this is the most difficult of the new yoga techniques. I put it on the routine that allows you to feel its benefit without wearing you out too much to finish the routine. However, you can always change these positions to fit your lifestyle and the order of the poses only matters to you.

Chapter 9: Standing Forward Fold (Bowing)

If you have any chronic hip or legs problems, this particular pose might not be suitable for you. Interestingly, you can do this same pose while seated.

Do you remember your basic training in proper lifting practices in the workplace? They always tell you to lift with your knees. Since you're not going to lift anything other than your own body weight with this pose, you can throw out that workplace directive because it contradicts lifting.

From a relaxed upright standing position, feet directly under your shoulders, you want to exhale and slowly hinge your hips so you are tilting forward. You want to bend at the knees enough to allow your body to fold onto itself. The final outcome of this exercise is the ability to place the palms of your hands on the floor.

It may seem unobtainable in the beginning of your exercise routine, but if you are diligent and keep practicing these yoga poses, you will see that eventually you can reach the floor from an upright position. Make sure to not put too much stress on your knees. Often people want to keep the knees in a locked position. Check with any physical therapist and they will assure you that maintaining locked knees during any exercise routine is not good for the longevity of your knees health.

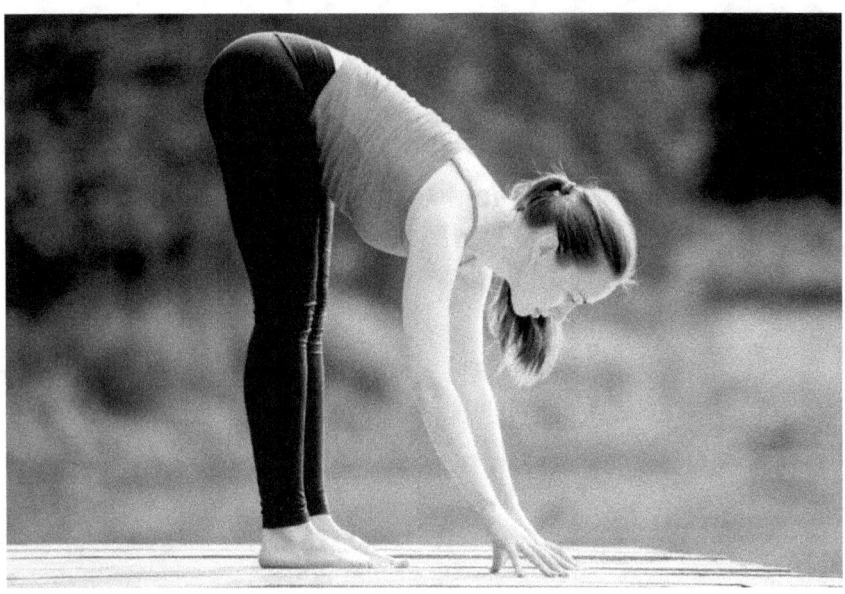

As you fold yourself forward, reaching for the floor, you should feel your spine stretching. If you can keep your head down, your arms directly over your ears, you can feel the tension on the back of your legs. Work this position in a manner that is constant, that is to not repeat folding, but to just press yourself forward one time. If you are breathing correctly, every time you exhale you can feel your body deepen into the stretch.

By the end of this pose, you should be able to, at least, brush the floor with your fingertips. Eventually, you will get the palms of your hands on the floor mat. Every breath will press your belly into your thighs.

When you have had enough of this pose, hold it until you feel the maximum benefit, and roll your body upward evenly and slowly. If you force yourself upright too fast you can get lightheaded. Roll your spine upward and gain a fully erect standing position. You should find you are facing forward, arms at your sides, and ready to complete your yoga exercise with the final pose.

Chapter 10: Child's Pose (Back to the Beginning)

If you decide to do all of the listed yoga poses, I recommend doing them in small doses. If you have any problems with weight or joint pain, you may find that afterward your body is crying out for some relaxation. As before, just take your time and remember to breathe. Any and all of these poses can be done in any order. The fluidity of the yoga poses, moving from one pose to the next, will likely become part of the routine.

This last pose, the Child's Pose is something that can be done at the beginning or end of your cycling yoga poses. I find at the end I like to be back on the mat and stretching out fully to get the maximum benefit of the exercises. At the end, I wanted something easy and found that I was out of breath. The Child's Pose helped me feel like I had concluded something significant.

Much like it sounds, the Child's Pose is something that likely all of us had done in adolescence. It helps me really stretch out my back. If I do it right I can feel vertebra popping back into place. As you sit on the mat you are actually sitting on your feet. Naturally your feet will want to turn inward to spread out your body weight evenly. If you have the strength, this is a good test you can work into your routine. What you want to eventually attain is the ability to sit on your feet with your ankles on the floor and the back of your toes against the mat. It sounds more complicated than it really is. When you feel it stretch your ankles and hips, you will understand that it's worth the tension in the lower extremities.

Begin by kneeling on the mat. Place your hands on your hips and breathe deeply. Slowing raise and lower your head, maintaining rigid shoulders. Allow your head to move on your neck without using your shoulders to help your head turn up and down. Slowly lift your head up so your chin is high in the air. Then lower your head so your chin touches your chest. You are maintaining a position on your feet and breathing accordingly.

Then from facing forward, turn your head to the left and to the right. Attempt to keep your shoulders straight, hands on your hips as you achieve this. You will feel your upper spine and shoulders want to help turn your head. By keeping your shoulders fixed you give your spine the opportunity to use some of the muscles that haven't been stretched in a long time; if you're like me.

After you have done this for five to ten breaths, you can slide your hands along your things and down to the mat in front of you. Press your upper body forward, sliding your hands along your legs and eventually on the floor. As you lower your head and shoulders, and allow your upper body to naturally roll forward.

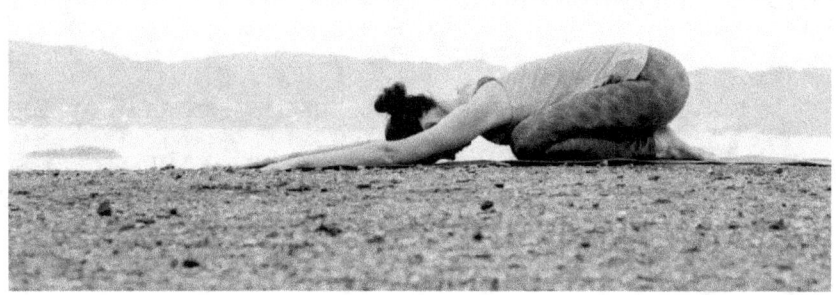

Sliding your hands along the floor, extend your arms straight, press your chest against your things as tight as you can comfortably. If you do this right, your face will be forward on the floor, your arms will be out straight on the mat and the weight of your body will be distributed across your thighs.

The idea you have here is as children we have the dexterity to twist ourselves into living pretzels. With some yoga poses, you can actually get into strange positions that may feel unnatural. Children don't usually bend themselves into impossible positions. Very young children will even sleep in a manner that is close to this yoga pose.

Try to hold this pose for some moments, your shoulders should be even with your ears, and your face should be straight to the floor; in line with your arms. If you can exhale deeply you will feel those vertebra loosen more and you can get deeper into the pose. It should feel natural, something the body remembers from its past.

I try to end my routine with this because it feels as if my body gets a better stretch as I exhale and press further into the pose.

Conclusion

I know I will never have rock-hard abdominal muscles. I'm a realist, I'm pragmatic. I understand that if I want to make more changes in my daily routine to get those glistening biceps and washboard abs, I'll need to buckle down and really focus on another routine. If I could afford an on-call nutritionist to serve all my meals, I likely would already be physically fit and wouldn't have worried about sharing this routine with anyone. I am comfortable with who I am. I am comfortable with how my life is going. I am comfortable with my current weight, waistline, and outlook on the rest of my life. Much like yoga, I will continue to practice living until I master it.

Yoga isn't for everyone, it is an acquired taste. It takes discipline and energy to work. I can't say that this little book will help lift you off the couch. I had an eye – opening experience that worked for me in a profound and enlightening way. I had no idea that I suffered from depression when I began practicing yoga. I knew I was overweight, obese even, but I suppose I had convinced myself that I was okay with how I looked until I wasn't any longer.

I can sleep through the night. If there is one thing to take away from this book, at least, stop drinking coffee late at night. Or stop drinking any caffeinated products that can disrupt the few precious hours you allow yourself to be selfish. Sleep is the one place you should have all to yourself. Yoga as a form of meditation is great, but in my opinion, it will never replace a comfortable mattress and a good night's sleep.

Yoga can change your life; if you let it happen. You may not get all the poses, all the stretching, or memorize the eight poses that I have covered in this book. However, I believe there will be something exciting and memorable in trying to achieve these specialized stances and poses. You may not be able to do it every day but try. It will surprise you how fast your day will open up when you either start or end your day with these few simple yoga poses. To allow yourself a perfect mind and body experience means to make time to allow it to happen.

When I started my yoga routine I weighed 289lbs, had a 44" waist, and a very unhealthy mind and body. After a few months, I felt better. I had more energy and a better sleep schedule. After a year, when I had lost over 100lbs and was down to a 36" waist, I knew I was onto something special. I understood that I had at least mastered my willpower to have a better outlook on life.

It begins hard, trust me, I know. But above all, remember the one constant in the millennia that yoga has been around: just *breathe...*